The Modern Guide to Vaping

Written by Craig Dunn

@crayfishx

www.vapingbook.info

Table of Contents

Disclaimer

Although every effort has been made by the author to ensure the information in this book was correct at the time of publication, the author does not assume any liability to any party for any loss, damage, disruption or injury caused by errors or omissions, whether such errors or omissions result from negligence, accident or any other cause.

All product and company names are trademarks or registered trademarks of their respective holders. Use of them does not imply any affiliation with or endorsement by them.

Introduction

There is such a huge range of product choices and styles associated with vaping that it can be a very daunting prospect for someone who is looking to make the shift from smoking to vaping. Even helpful Internet forums can appear to be full of people talking in a foreign language with numerous cryptic acronyms and strange terms like *squonking* and *dripping*, With this book I intend to remove some of the mystery around vaping and help you start your own journey. Starting with an explanation of the basic components of vaping covering the multitude of different device types on the market, and then exploring more advanced vaping techniques and practices such as building your own device components.

I hope this book serves as a useful guide through the fascinating world of vaping and help you find your own way.

My Journey

I still remember it well. I was fourteen years old, sitting at home with my grandmother who was a lifelong smoker. As she reached over to the coffee table for her leather cigarette pouch and silver lighter she observed my face, my eyes slowly tracking every movement of her hands and a visible yearning in my expression.

 She placed a cigarette between her lips and lit it, as she took a deep breath and let the smoke out she continued studying me before reaching again for her cigarette pouch. Without any hesitation she opened the pack, leaned over slightly and extended out her hand. "Would you like a cigarette?" she asked.

You may be forgiven for thinking this was a rather irresponsible thing for a grandparent to ask a teenager, but she knew me well. She knew just from looking at my face that I had smoked before, and in her mind she would rather I did something out in the open in front of her than behind her back. She was right, I had tried smoking already, and I liked it.

After recovering from the initial shock of my grandmother offering me a cigarette, I nervously said yes and reached out and took a single cigarette from her pack. Still trembling with nerves and disbelief at what I was doing in front of her, I clumsily lit the cigarette and we sat in silence for the next few minutes, enjoying for the first time the experience of smoking together.

Little did I know how much that moment would shape the rest of my life, fast forward twenty five years and I look back at over two decades of being a smoker, well over half of my lifetime. I had tried numerous times to quit with varying degrees of success. I once went cold turkey and gave up smoking completely. That lasted for six months before a stressful situation re-ignited my desire to smoke to a point I couldn't say no anymore.

I resented cold turkey. Despite knowing the damage that smoking tobacco was doing to my body, and as a result my life expectancy, I couldn't stop. Smoking was my crutch, my friend and my support. The desire to stop smoking was there, but nothing could replace my old friend, the little companion I had held between my fingers for so many years.

I struggled with all the conventional ways to quit smoking. Nicotine replacement therapies (NRT) such as patches and gum were just useless for me, because whilst they were feeding my chemical addiction to nicotine, smoking for me was far more than that. It was a process, a routine and a habit, and all of the therapies available at the time would take that away and rob me of what I had come to depend on for years.

My journey with vaping began nine years ago, when I spotted an advertisement for a new product, an electronic cigarette. It promised to offer all the joy and satisfaction of smoking with none of the health risks associated with burning tobacco.   This revolutionary product seemed like a dream come true, finally a way I could continue to enjoy the pleasures of being a smoker but be able to silence that little voice in the back of my head constantly telling me that I'm slowly killing myself.

This first foray into the world of vaping did not go well. I was filled with excitement when I opened up the newly delivered package and put together a small device resembling a cigarette. I followed the instructions, inserted a little cartridge that came with the device and tried this entirely new form of "smoking" for the first time. As the little blue light at the end of the device lit up when I dragged in a lungful of air and slowly exhaled I came to a startling realization, it was disgusting. It left a rancid taste in my nasal cavities and my mouth and in no way lived up to the expectations I had set. It was clear that this was not something that I was going to even remotely enjoy and would never come close to helping me quit smoking cigarettes. My newly purchased e-cigarette promptly found its way to living at the bottom of a drawer and I continued on my destructive path of tobacco smoking.

My journey did not end there however. Fortunately creativity and innovation began to flourish in the industry and before long a new generation of more advanced devices began to appear on the market such as refillable electronic cigarettes that allowed you to chose from a wide variety of flavored liquids. This second generation of electronic cigarettes was a vast improvement and before long I was drawn back into the fascinating world of vaping.

I found myself vaping regularly, sometimes for long periods up to weeks or months, but I always seemed destined to return to smoking tobacco. For the last year or two of being a smoker I was using both electronic cigarettes and smoking conventional tobacco. This helped me for a long time cut down my smoking but I was finding it hard to make that hard switch, to say goodbye once and for all to something that had defined me for so long, to be an ex-smoker.

There were two important drivers for me that eventually lead to me switching full time to vaping and quitting smoking. I was thirty nine years old and I had convinced myself that I should make a change when I turn forty. Forty is just a number but for me it was important, it was a mental cut off point, a place in my life where I needed to think about the future and my health as I age. There is also scientific research suggesting the health benefits and life expectancy gained by quitting before the age of forty are significant.

The second motivation for me was my son, then aged two. Not only did I not want him growing up exposed to tobacco smoke but I also wanted to ensure that I gave myself the best possible chance to see as much of his life as possible and be there as he becomes a man and makes his own way into the world. It was time to make a real effort.

I am a regular traveler for work and for some time I had realized that I could easily go up to a week without a cigarette when I was on the road, relying only on my electronic cigarette to get me through the week. I decided initially that I would try and continue with this pattern. When I went away on trips I would not bring a packet of cigarettes with me and I would simply tell myself that I was going to try not to buy any until I returned. After a couple of months of successfully not smoking on my business trips I decided it was time to tackle my smoking habit at home. This was by far the biggest challenge for me. Sitting on my terrace in the evening sipping a cold beer went hand in hand with smoking a cigarette, as did visiting my local bar. These were trigger situations that I knew would be hard to endure, but if I was going to finally be able to break the powerful hold that tobacco held over me, I knew I had to face this head on.

I decided from the beginning that I would not announce my grand plan to friends and family, even to my wife I just said that I am going to try and smoke less at home. For me, announcing to the world that you are going to stop smoking makes it a challenge, and fear of failure would lead me right back to smoking. I didn't want the pressure of knowing that if I smoked another cigarette I would have failed. Instead I just set out my intentions to smoke less. One morning I sat with a coffee and used my electronic cigarette instead of lighting up. That first day I decided to see if I could go the whole day without smoking, and I did. The next day I repeated the process, again without making any commitments or promises.

During this time I researched in depth all of the different vaping options out there. The vaping world had moved on in leaps and bounds since those disappointing devices I had tried years before and flourished into a multi billion dollar industry. I discovered there was a plethora of different types devices, methods and styles of vaping. I experimented with many of the various different types of electronic cigarettes and flavor types. It took time to fully explore the huge variety of options available and to identify what I liked and disliked. A turning point for me came one night sitting on my terrace vaping a lovely caramel flavored liquid in a device I had purchased that week. As I exhaled an impressive cloud of vapor, I sat back and realized *"I enjoy this more than smoking!"*. That was the moment for me when I knew that I hadn't just found something to help me stay off cigarettes, I had found something better than smoking.

Vaping for me became far more than just a way to quit smoking. I began to embrace it and discovered a whole new hobby. I started using rebuildable atomizers and mixing my own juices. Not only has vaping saved precious years of my life but it has also given me an enjoyable, albeit sometimes expensive pastime.

This was my personal journey, yours will be very different.

Introduction to Vaping

History

Vaping as we know it today may seem like a very recent evolution, but the origins of vaping go back further than you might think. In fact, it can be dated all the way back to 1927 when a man named Joseph Robinson filed a patent in the United States for a device that could be used to heat and vaporize liquid to be inhaled by the user.

The proposed device specified in the original patent application shared many design features with a modern day electronic cigarette. Robinson's device was not an electronic cigarette however, he intended for his invention to be used for the administration of certain medical compounds. His patent was approved but the product was never launched.

Several decades later in 1963 it was Herbert A. Gilbert who invented what could be regarded the oldest relative of the modern day electronic cigarette. Gilbert patented his device as a smokeless alternative to smoking cigarettes that operated by using a wicking method to provide liquid to a heating element that allowed the liquid to be vaporized and inhaled. His vision was never realized however, at a time when smoking was prolific and the dangers of smoking were little known. Although Gilbert prototyped and distributed his device, the concept never took on and eventually his patent lay dormant for years until eventually expiring.

The modern day story of vaping began in the early 2000s. A Chinese pharmacist and medical researcher named Hon Lik developed the first electronic cigarette to make it to the mainstream market. Hon Lik had watched his father pass away from a smoking related illness and himself had struggled with a long battle to give up smoking. He claims that a dream in which he was drowning in water which then became vapor enabling him to breath lead him to to design his invention. In 2006, Lik released his first product as an alternative to smoking tobacco, a device that used an ultrasonic component to vaporize a liquid mixture containing nicotine. Hon Lik's innovative product marked the birth of the vaping revolution as we know it today.

Before long, a pair of brothers in the United Kingdom named Umer and Tariq Sheikh built upon this idea and developed what became known as a cartomizer and later advanced that technology to produce a tank style system known as a clearomizer, a design that many of the modern electronic cigarettes on sale today derive from.

In recent years vaping has exploded in popularity saving millions of people world wide from a lifetime of smoking harmful tobacco products.

Vaping has lead to a multi billion dollar industry and developed into a sub culture of society. Vaping exhibitions are seeing year on year increases in popularity. Internet forums are packed with people sharing their experiences and helping people in the vaping community and vape shops seem to be springing up on every street corner in some cities.

Health and Vaping

The important distinction that separates smoking from vaping is that with tobacco smoking, many chemicals are released by combustion, or burning, of a product, and a smoker inhales smoke produced from the burning of the materials within the cigarette. It has been proven that this smoke contains many hundreds of chemicals, a vast majority of them being hazardous to human health. The practice of vaping does not involve any combustion, merely a heating of liquid and the contents are delivered to the user in a vapor form.

There are varying viewpoints on the health risks associated with vaping. Very few people would argue that vaping poses absolutely no risk, and because vaping has really only existed for a decade or so, and the devices we use have changed so rapidly over an even shorter space of time there are few scientific studies able to research the longer term effects of vaping. Bearing in mind that most vapers are ex-smokers for whom, if it were not for vaping, would almost certainly continue smoking tobacco products, I think the question should be how safe vaping is in comparison to smoking of cigarettes.

I have decided not to write specifically about health issues in any great detail in this book. I am not in any way a trained medical professional therefore I feel this is a subject matter that I am not qualified to write about in an informative way.

I can however share a personal experience, one not based in any way on scientific knowledge. Since finally making the permanent switch to vaping from tobacco smoking I have felt fantastic. Gone is the intense morning cough that would sound out throughout the house as I hacked up vast quantities of gunk from my lungs minutes after getting out of bed, as is the shortness of breath by walking briskly half a mile down the road. I feel healthier now in my forties than I did in my early thirties.

I encourage you to do your own research of what reputable scientific institutes are saying and make your own informed choice of what you choose to put into your body. Remember that the Internet is not the most objective of mediums, this is the same place where plenty of people believe that the Earth is flat and is controlled by lizard like reptilian beings. You must question the authenticity of reports online and separate unfounded opinion based science from research conducted by well respected scientific bodies who don't have a political or idealogical agenda to push.

My personal sources of information that I trust include Public Health England who have stated that based on current research they consider vaping is likely to be 95% safer than smoking, and Cancer Research UK who back those claims. As someone who knows full well the alternative road that waits for me if I didn't vape, I'll take those odds!

Ultimately it's your body, and your choice.

E-Cigarettes

When you first step into the world of vaping, it can be very daunting to navigate the complex variety of differing types of electronic cigarettes and accessories on the market. From small plastic tubes that closely resemble cigarettes to metal boxes with baffling LED displays and glass tanks sitting on top. In this chapter we will look at the main types of device and explain the differences between them.

People have very differing reasons for wanting to vape and those reasons heavily influence the type of vaping devices that are more suitable for them. In this book we will explore the more common types of vaping devices from entry level to the more advanced and complex setups.

It's important to remember that we are all different. A common theme in this book is to point out that there are no answers, and that is because there is no one type of vape that works for everyone, everything in vaping comes down to what you like, not what is considered better. There is no obligation to always seek to move to a more advanced style of vaping, the most important thing is that you find a method of vaping that you are comfortable with.   I do however encourage you to experiment, as I did, to try a variety of vaping setups until you find what ultimately satisfies you

The practice of vaping is, fundamentally, using a personal device to inhale vapor generated by heating a liquid into the lungs. The liquid used in this process usually, but not necessarily, contains nicotine and some flavorings. Typically the vapor is thick enough to be visible in the air upon exhaling, re-producing for many the sensation and experience of smoking a tobacco cigarette.

All electronic cigarette devices share some common characteristics. Although designs and capabilities differ enormously across different makes and models, the basic function of an electronic cigarette remains the same. Most electronic cigarettes contain the same basic components. First there is a compartment or tank to store a small amount of liquid. The liquid is then soaked up by some kind of wicking method, often cotton based, to a wire coil. A battery power source is then used to heat the coil containing the soaked cotton, because the cotton is wet it does not burn and instead heats the liquid within it to a temperature sufficient enough to vaporize. The released vapor is then inhaled by the user.

Although all electronic cigarettes fundamentally perform the same function, there are many factors which need considering when deciding on which type of setup is suitable for you, and in this chapter we will look at some of the main types of e-cigarettes and what they offer.

Cig-a-likes

The most basic form of device available on the market today are known as cig-a-likes. They are so named primarily because they often closely resemble a conventional cigarette in the way they are designed. Often they are white with yellow tips, and some models even have small colored lights on the tips that activate when the user inhales further attempting to recreate the exact experience of smoking for the user.

Cig-a-likes are often made up of two components, the main body of the device housing a small internal rechargeable battery to power the device, and disposable cartridges that provide a liquid containing nicotine and a small element to heat the liquid and produce vapor. The liquid in the cartridge is typically soaked in a polyfill material enabling it to be carried to the heating element.

Users of these types of devices are usually not full time vapers or ex-smokers, simply because the level of vapor production and flavor often falls short of satisfying the user. I would not recommend you start with cig-a-likes if your intention is to quit using tobacco and make a permanent switch to vaping. That said, like everything in the vaping world, personal preference differs from person to person and some people do successfully move from smoking to vaping using cig-a-like type devices. Cig-a-likes are however popular with people just looking to experiment with the idea of electronic cigarettes, or for smokers who may wish to have an alternative method of smoking in situations where are unable to smoke conventional tobacco.

Pods

Vaping pods are a relatively new addition to the vaping world. They are a popular entry level device for vapers looking for a no frills, uncomplicated vaping experience but wish for something a little more advanced than the very basic cig-a-like options. Pods come in all sorts of shapes, the difference between these systems and other more advanced devices that we will go on to discuss is that they use a bespoke pod that contains e-liquid and fits onto the main unit. Some pods are refillable but the majority are disposable and are sold in a variety of basic flavors.

Pod systems are superior to cig-a-likes as they generally offer better battery life and the pods themselves that contain the e-liquid and heating element to create vapor offer a more satisfying flavorful vaping experience than their cig-a-like cousins.

Some pod systems, in particular one brand known as *JUUL*, have been the subject of some controversy, mainly in the United States where many people claim they are responsible for a recent upsurge in vaping among teenagers. This is partly due to their availability, low cost and the fact they can be carried and used very discreetly.

Vape Pens

A more advanced device commonly used by new vapers is the pen style vaporizer. These entry level devices are cylindrically shaped and typically made up of two sections. The first section houses an internal rechargeable battery and has a firing button. The battery component connects to a small tank containing the liquid. Within the tank there is a small component known as an atomizer which contains the wire coil that is heated to produce vapor from the liquid contained in the tank when the user presses the fire button. The atomizer usually has some kind of wicking method made from a cotton based material to soak up the liquid in the tank and carry it to the heating coil.

These types of e-cigarettes allow the user to refill the liquid reservoir of the device. Liquids are available in a huge range of flavors and nicotine strengths, meaning this type of system gives the user a lot more choice and control over their vaping experience than offered by the cig-a-like or pod alternatives.

The origins of vaping pens began with the clearomizer. A clearomizer is a disposable thin cylindrical tank made of clear plastic that connects to a battery unit. E-liquid is added to the tank by unscrewing the top mouth-piece and adding liquid directly into to the reservoir area. The e-liquid is then soaked up into a small atomizer unit by wicks that extend from the atomizer and float in the tank.

The biggest brand name of clearomizer style devices is called Ego, or Ego-C. Although a brand specific to a particular manufacturer, the term Ego is often used in the vaping community to refer to clearomizer devices in general, a bit like how the brand Hoover became synonymous with other vacuum cleaners not made by Hoover Inc. These types of devices are aimed mainly at people new to vaping. They can be very effective in helping users curtail their tobacco usage or quit smoking altogether. Often, but not always, new vapers will use clearomizers to familiarize themselves with the practice of vaping and eventually find themselves moving on to slightly more advanced kits in order to maximize the experience delivered from vaping and give them more choice and convenience in how they want to vape.

Recent years have seen a progression in innovation around vaping pens and the emergence of new products in the marketplace that offer more versatile features than the basic Ego style clearomizers, such as the ability to adjust the power level delivered to the atomizer allowing the user to opt for a cooler or warmer vape depending on their preference. They are cylindrical tubes, often thicker and more durable than more basic Ego style models and have higher capacity battery and a sturdier permanent tank usually made out of metal and glass containing the atomizer.

With usage, the coil and the wicking material of the atomizer contained in the tank becomes less effective, which can eventually lead to the atomizer burning out, rendering it ineffective and unable to produce quality vapor. When a coil is no longer functioning optimally, typically after about two weeks of use depending on the model, but this can vary greatly depending on several factors that we will discuss later, the atomizer component of the tank can be removed and replaced with a new one, or in the case of clearomizers, the entire tank section of the vaping pen can be replaced relatively cheaply.

Mods

In the earlier days of vaping there was a limited number of products on the market and most were fairly low powered devices. Many more experienced vapers were seeking ways to maximize their experience and increase the vapor production from their atomizers. To do this they required more power to be delivered to the atomizer than was currently possible with the range of conventional devices on the market. This lead to the emergence of a new practice known as *modding*. Hobbyists began experimenting with alternative ways of producing power from larger batteries and modifying other electronic items such as high powered flashlights to build their own homemade devices capable of firing atomizers at higher power to deliver a more satisfying vaping experience. These devices were commonly referred to as mods.

These days there are still pockets of hobbyists who continue to invent their own vaporizing devices either from scratch or by transforming other electrical devices, but the term mod these days usually refers to the power supply and control component of any mid-range to advanced vaping device and is typically commercially mass manufactured.

Mid range to advanced vaping devices typically consist of two main parts, a mod and a tank. I will go on to discuss tanks in much more detail, but they perform the function of storing e-liquid and delivering it to the heating coil to be vaporized.

A mod is generally referred to as a device containing a battery power source that is responsible for delivering power to a tank in order for it to vaporize e-liquid.

The vast majority of mods and tanks across all manufacturers share a common connection standard known as a 510 thread. This means, unlike all-in-one devices and pens, users are free to mix and match different mods and tanks from different vendors to find a setup that offers them the best solution for their vaping needs.

As with all things vaping, there are a wide variety of different types of mods on the market and it's important to choose the right type of mod to suit your vaping needs. There are two distinct classes of mods, regulated and mechanical.

Regulated Mods

Regulated mods refer to a type of mod that has electrical circuitry and controls to allow the user to control the amount of power delivered by the mod to the atomizer. They are the most commonly used mods on the market by both beginner and advanced vapers.

Styles of regulated mods vary from cylindrical chambers to chunky rectangular devices often referred to as *box mods*. They typically have a 510 thread connection at the top for connecting a tank, a fire button to operate the device and controls for adjusting the power that is delivered to atomizer. Most will have a small LED screen for displaying information such as power status.

More advanced regulated mods offer many more features to allow for alternative forms of vaping such as temperature controlled mode, where the mod will try and automatically drive the correct amount of power to maintain a specific temperature in the coil when fired.

Regulated mods can have either an internal battery rechargeable by a USB connection or a use external lithium-ion batteries. The decision of whether or not to use an external or internal battery device is important. Many people who vape daily choose to use an external battery solution as it allows them to carry spare batteries to ensure they are capable of uninterrupted vaping throughout the day. This is an important factor if you are vaping to completely quit a heavy smoking habit and worry that waiting for a number of hours for your mod to recharge will return you to tobacco smoking.

Other larger mods can take two or even three external batteries. These more advanced mods cater for different styles of vaping that we will go on to explore later in this book.

Mechanical Mods

Mechanical mods, often called simply *'mech mods'*, are a type of mod that is   similar in function to a regulated mod but constructed entirely out of mechanical parts.

Mechanical mods do not contain any electronic circuit boards or chips and are operated by a fire button that creates a physical circuit connecting the battery and the wire coil in the atomizer.

Many advanced vapers prefer mechanical mods over regulated mods because of their durability due to the absence of potentially fragile circuit boards and other electronic components. The electronic circuitry in a regulated device not only offers the ability to control the amount of power drawn from the battery and delivered to the atomizer, but also gives various levels of safety protection. These features are not present in a mechanical mod. The power drawn from the battery is dependent on the coil wire that connects the positive and negative ends of the circuit and without the proper knowledge of batteries and electronics you risk seriously stressing your batteries to the point of failure.

Mechanical mods also offer no protection against hard shorting a battery, where the positive end of the battery makes contact with the negative end via a conductive material within the device.   Furthermore regulated devices have reverse polarity protection which prevents failure if you insert your battery the wrong way around, whereas a mechanical mod has no such protection. All of these scenarios with a mechanical mod can not only destroy your device but potentially be extremely dangerous and risk serious injury.

That is not to say that anyone choosing to use a mechanical mod is doing anything inherently dangerous, many people vape mechanical mods perfectly safely, but it is very important to understand that these are people with experience of battery safety and electronics who fully understand how their devices work. If you are reading this book as a beginner, I would strongly advise starting with a regulated device and avoiding mechanical mods until you are fully comfortable and knowledgeable about it.

Coils

A coil the wire element within the atomizer that the cotton is passed through to draw in the e-liquid. When you fire your e-cigarette it's the coil that heats up to vaporize the liquid and deliver your vaping experience. Most coils are built into a small closed device called an atomizer head along with the wicking material and are housed inside a chamber, or tank, to hold the liquid.

After some use, the coil can start to drop in performance and begin to deliver dry or burnt tasting hits when vaping. This is usually a sign that the coil has reached the end of it' life and requires replacing. With most tank systems the coil is easily removable by unscrewing the base of the unit allowing you to replace it with a new one.

It's hard to say how long a coil will last in general, it depends on many factors including the frequency in which you vape, the power setting you use and the type of e-juice you are using. Coils can last anywhere from a couple of days to two months.

There are some things you can do to help prolong the life of your coil and avoid having to change it excessively. If you find your coils are burning out very regularly it may be that you are using your e-cigarette at a higher power level than is suitable for the coil in the atomizer, in this case you can try adjusting the wattage level down and work up very slowly until you find a comfortable vaping experience that keeps your coils going for longer.

One of the most common questions among new vapers using variable wattage device is what power level should they vape at. Whilst there are some rules of thumb that can put you in a rough ballpark, there is no formula or chart that can tell you what power level you should be using. Using less power will deliver a slightly cooler vape with less vapor, which is how some people like to vape, and others prefer a warmer, denser vape produced by using their device at a higher power setting.

A lot of coils have a recommended power range in watts printed on the side. These ratings can often be inflated in order to make the coil more attractive to the cloud chaser. I have often found the optimum power setting for a particular coil to be far below the recommended range. It's better to start off at a lower power setting and slowly work up in small increments until you find a level that delivers the level of flavor and vapor production that satisfies you and not always pay attention to the recommended wattage claimed by the manufacturer.

When firing your device, the cotton surrounding the coils must be soaked in e-liquid or you risk burning the cotton, which not only results in an unpleasant harsh, burnt taste, but will dramatically shorten the life of your coil as burning is irreversible. To avoid this, always make sure that your tank is sufficiently full of e-liquid when vaping.

Similarly, when installing a new coil it is recommended that you *prime* the coil prior to first use. Priming a coil involves placing a small amount of e-liquid onto the inside of the atomizer where the cotton meets the metal coil to ensure that it is adequately soaked before firing it for the first time. Since atomizers draw liquid into the the coils slowly, failing to prime your coils could easily result in no liquid reaching the coils when you first fire your device and your cotton could instantly burn and destroy the new coil.   When priming, you should be aiming to wet the cotton, not soak the entire interior of the atomizer with e-liquid as this could have the opposite effect and flood your coil.

Flooding is when too much liquid enters the center of the atomizer and the coil is surrounded by a pool of liquid, rather than just wet cotton. This can result in gurgling, spitting of hot juice into your mouth and create a very unpleasant vape. Coils can flood for a variety of reasons, including juice that is too thin, a faulty or expiring atomizer or by over priming the coil as we have discussed.

If this all sounds very complicated, don't worry, it won't take long before you get used to your coils – even experienced vapers need to experiment a little with a new type of coil until the find what works for them.

Power and Ohms

The main difference between different types of coils is the optimal power setting that can be used to obtain the best vaping experience. The level of power appropriate for a particular coil is largely decided by a factor called *resistance.* The resistance of a coil determines, in basic terms, the amount of difficulty presented for current to pass through it and is measured using a unit known as ohms, represented with the Greek Omega symbol Ω.

There are many online resources dedicated to in depth explanations of ohms and how it relates to voltage and amperage, in this book I don't want to get too bogged down in the science of it, and I want to be able to inform total beginners without getting into an electronics lesson. But we'll discuss the points relevant to vaping.

A coil will often have its ohms measurement printed on the side, and most modern mods are capable of reading and displaying the ohms measurement of the coil, which can sometimes be a tiny bit higher or lower than the advertised resistance. But what does this mean?

The most basic explanation of resistance is, the higher the number of ohms, the more resistance the coil has. That is to say, it is more difficult for current to flow through the coil. Conversely, the lower numbers indicate that there is less resistance and the coil is capable of easily passing more current.

What this means in the context of vaping is that higher resistance coils, those less capable of passing large amounts of current, require less power to heat the e-liquid in the coil. While this may be great for extending your battery life, it also restricts the amount of vapor that can be produced to a degree.

Lower resistance coils have more mass and are usually capable of vaporizing more e-liquid. Many people like to vape at lower resistances in order to produce more vapor and a denser, fuller vaping experience. In order to achieve this however they generally require more power and therefore will drain more from the devices battery.

It's important to realize that, unlike the wattage used to power your coils, resistance it not something you can configure or adjust using your mod. It is a physical characteristic of the wire used in your coil determined by its mass and volume.

If you're struggling with this concept, think of a hosepipe versus a drinking straw. Let's imagine that you are the battery, and the water is the electrical current. With both of these we are capable of putting them to our lips and blowing water through them. The drinking straw requires a very small amount of effort from you to pass water through at an optimal rate but the amount of water, or current, that passes through the straw is minimal. The hosepipe however is capable of passing a great deal more water. But if we use the same effort to pass water through the hosepipe as we did with the drinking straw we won't achieve anywhere near the optimal level of throughput, so to compensate for this we need to exert considerably more energy.

This is the same relationship your batteries have with your coils, in order to optimally fire a lower resistance coil to achieve a throughput great enough to heat our e-liquid we have to consider the power needed based on the resistance of the coil.

Sub-Ohming

If you've spent a little time around the vaping community online you would have probably come across the phrase *sub-ohming* by now. Put simply, 'to sub-ohm' refers to vaping at a resistance of 1.0Ω or lower. Some vaping kits come with coils measuring a resistance of 1.4-1.8Ω, although they can go even higher. At the other end of the scale vapers who are seeking a much denser, cloudier experience often chose to use coils anywhere from 0.4Ω down to 0.1Ω in order to vape at much higher wattages than would be suitable on higher resistance coils. Regulated mods normally have an upper and lower limit of coil resistance that they are able to fire so if you're looking at seriously sub-ohming you should make sure you have a device capable of firing at that range.

Although we use the term sub-ohming to describe vaping at any resistance below 1.0Ω, there is nothing that special about this number when it comes to vaping – it's just a scale, there is not a lot of difference between vaping at 1.0Ω and vaping at 0.9Ω.

Sub-ohming used to be the practice of the vaping elite, which is probably why it earned its own verb. Several years ago factory made coils were generally only 1.2Ω or higher, so people with mechanical mods started building their own components to achieve resistance levels in the sub-ohm ranges to deliver a more robust, intense vape by drawing more power from the battery. Regulated mods however are able to control how much power is drawn from the battery making the ohms rating of the coil a less important factor in achieving a fuller vape, however for those wishing to vape at very high wattages, using a coil of a lower resistance or sub-ohm offers the best performance. Devices over recent years have advanced and even entry to mid-range e-cigarettes now pack more power with many sporting dual batteries, the vast majority of even beginner kits these days will use coils in the sub-ohm range.

When vaping using coils built to sub-ohm resistance levels it is important to be aware that in order to fire coils of very low resistance sufficiently to vaporize the liquid effectively you are going to need to drive more power to your coil by increasing the amount of watts you vape at. This increase in wattage will place extra strain on your batteries and it's important to understand how to ensure you are vaping within the safe stress limits of the battery you are using. We will discuss this and other battery safety issues later in this book.

Vaping Style

Mouth-to-lung and Direct-to-lung

Most vapers fall into one of two categories that defines the primary method of vaping they enjoy. The first is *mouth-to-lung,* often referred to as 'MTL'. This method of vaping is more reflective of the act of smoking tobacco and involves drawing vapor into your mouth and holding it there a short time before inhaling into your lungs. Because of its similarity to cigarette smoking, this is the method most often employed by new vapers who are moving from tobacco products to vaping.

The second vaping style is called *direct to lung,* or 'DL'. Using this method, the vaper will inhale the vapor released by the atomizer directly into their lungs by simply breathing in whilst applying and firing the device. This style of vapor inhalation is more similar to that of asthma inhalers than of cigarettes. Generally speaking direct to lung vaping is capable of generating much fuller clouds of vapor, although many say that flavor can be more intense using the mouth to lung method.

Finding the right vaping style for you is very much a personal choice. Whilst most people do start off with an MTL style, not everyone moves on to direct lung vaping. Some people even bounce between direct-lung and mouth-to-lung throughout the day, opting for a more discreet vape when out and about and cloud chasing by night in their own homes. It all boils down to the individual. But the style of vaping you enjoy will be an important factor in determining which tank to use.

Cloud Chasers and Flavor Chasers

The second notable distinction between vapers is their desire to either focus on the flavor of the e-liquid they are vaping or the density and quantity of the vapor clouds they produce. Over time these different vaping goals have resulted in people normally falling into one of two categories of either *flavor chasers* or *cloud chasers*.

Generally speaking, but not always, one often comes at the expense of the other.

Many people more concerned with flavor than the level of vapor production often opt for a mouth-to-lung style device whereas some vapers will opt for larger more powerful devices capable of producing impressive clouds. Cloud chasers generally opt for direct to lung style vaping as this offers the maximum potential for vapor production, but also requires substantially more e-liquid.

Stealth Vaping

Stealth vaping is a term used to describe the act of vaping in the most discrete way. Normally this means selecting and tuning a vaporizer to be able to vape without producing noticeable clouds of vapor and sometimes using e-liquids that do not have a particularly detectable smell.

Different situations carry varying levels of social acceptance regarding where and when it is suitable to vape, and rapidly evolving policies in some establishments mean sometimes it is prohibited. Adjusting your vaping style depending on the immediate situation is commonplace among vapers.

I would class myself as firmly a cloud chasing, direct to lung style of vaper. However, although it's perfectly legal in my home country to vape at a bar or restaurant, I would quickly draw unwanted negative attention to my actions if I started filling my immediate surroundings with massive clouds, which would likely lead to a polite, or not so polite, request for me to cease vaping. In these circumstances I'll often opt for a more discreet stealthy style of vaping that I can enjoy without negatively impacting those around me.

E-Liquid

So far we've looked at various aspects of the hardware involved in vaping, but another key consideration to make when determining an optimal experience is the e-liquid that you use.

As electronic cigarettes first hit the mainstream market they were mostly in the form of Cig-a-like style devices with a disposable cartridge containing the e-liquid to vaporize. As I related earlier when discussing my own journey into the world of vaping, the taste of the liquid used was not pleasant, at least not for me.

The emergence of more advanced devices with refillable tank sections allowing the user to add their own liquid lead to another drive in innovation and creation in the vaping world, flavored e-liquid.

Out went the dull and unappealing taste of generic e-liquid and in came new and inventive flavors including strawberry, apple, banana, coffee and chocolate. As e-juice manufacturers have honed their craft, e-liquids have moved beyond the basic binary flavors and given rise to a plethora of complex and exotic recipes simulating the taste of everything from cinnamon and apple pie to bubble gum.

The range of flavors available now is simply huge with new recipes being developed all the time. Most flavors fall into one of a number of flavor profiles that might be preferred by the vaper, including fruits, sweets, custards and creams but the diversity of options in these profiles is seemingly unending. Much like food, the best flavors to vape are entirely down to individual preference, while one vaper may love strawberry jam donut flavor, another may hate it.

Finding the right flavors to suit you may take time. A recommended way to start exploring different flavor types is to first identify what flavor profile you enjoy most and then focus on that group of flavors trying different recipes until you find some that you enjoy more than others. Of course, many people vape a variety of flavors from different profiles even in the same day. I sometimes prefer a fruit based vape in the mornings and during the day, but with a beer in the evening I enjoy a sweeter experience such as butterscotch and cream.

People are often encouraged to be adventurous with food, trying new food groups and things that are sometimes out of their comfort zone. The same is true with vaping, don't assume what you won't enjoy until you've tried it. By experimenting and sampling all sorts of different flavors you will not only discover some wonderful recipes that you enjoy, but you'll have fun doing it.

Composition

The e-liquid we use for vaping is made up of a base mixture containing propylene glycol (PG) and vegetable glycerin (VG). Both of these ingredients are used very commonly in all sorts of consumable products from cough syrup to candy bars and ice creams. They are both odorless liquids that when heated produce a visible vapor. It is this base mix that gives vaping its clouds.

VG has a higher viscosity than PG meaning that the ratio of VG to PG in a particular e-liquid will determine the thickness of the resulting liquid is. Liquids of a very thick or thin consistency may not be suitable for some coils as either the cotton will not be able to soak up the liquid fast enough and result in dry or burnt hits, or conversely a very thin liquid might seep into the coils too quickly causing it to flood.

There are some other differences between the two liquids that make up the base mix. When heated, VG produces thicker and denser vapor than PG. Vapers who want to make large and impressive clouds tend to choose liquids higher in VG for this purpose.

PG on the other hand is largely responsible for delivering the throat hit sensation. Some people prefer a harsher throat hit to others whereas some people enjoy a smoother vaping experience with little or no throat hit. Choosing the right balance between PG and VG can help in finding the level of throat hit that is suitable for you.

Most e-liquid manufacturers will display the ratio of VG to PG on the product label. The three most common ratios are 50/50, where there is an equal amount of PG to VG, 70/30 which is a common baseline for a lot of vapers indicating the base mix is made up of 70% VG and 30% PG, and finally 80/20 which is popular with people who enjoy a higher VG mix and provides 80% VG and 20% PG.

VG and PG are both non toxic liquids and safe for human consumption, however some people do report a sensitivity or allergy to PG when vaporized. Those who find themselves sensitive to PG based mixes can opt to vape a mix very high in VG, or with no PG whatsoever.

Suspended within the base mix are the flavorings that make up the e-liquid recipe. Flavorings are usually made up of natural and artificial extracts and food additives that are safe for consumption. It's important that you only vape with flavorings that have explicitly been made for vaping. The chemical composition of some liquids can change substantially when heated and vaporized, just because something is safe to eat or drink does not automatically mean that it's safe for vaping.

Nicotine

The final ingredient found in e-liquid is nicotine. Since most vapers are current or ex-smokers and are using vaping to replace or reduce their tobacco usage, the vast majority of people use an e-liquid with nicotine. Using nicotine however is by no means a requirement and there are plenty of people who opt to vape without nicotine. For some people the habit and routine of smoking is harder to break than the chemical addiction to nicotine and they find themselves able to vape without nicotine but the act of vaping is enough to satisfy their habit and prevent them from returning to smoking tobacco.

Nicotine is an addictive substance and toxic in very high doses, although the levels found in e-liquids are not dangerous. It is a stimulant which means it does have some physiological side effects on your body, including raising your blood pressure and constricting blood vessels, however it is not the nicotine in conventional cigarettes that are attributed to heart disease and cancer. The majority of harm from smoking tobacco comes from the chemicals and tar released from the combustion of the materials and inhalation of smoke. Vaping does not burn any materials and therefore these harmful elements can be avoided giving the vaper a method of getting nicotine that is widely claimed to be much safer by magnitudes than doing so by inhaling the products of combustion.

E-liquids contain varying levels of nicotine. The strength of nicotine in an e-liquid mix is usually represented in milligrams per milliliter, or *mg/ml*. Often it is just written as a number followed by the letters *mg,* but this does not indicate the total amount of nicotine in the bottle. For example, a liquid displaying *6mg* has 6 milligrams of nicotine for every milliliter of liquid, meaning a 10ml bottle would contain 60mg of nicotine in total.

If you chose to vape with nicotine then you need to select the strength that best suits you. There are various factors to consider when determining what strength nicotine to select and a lot depends on your current circumstances.

People making the move from smoking to vaping in order to stop using tobacco products are recommended to start at a higher nicotine level and slowly work down. Failure to select a high enough nicotine level when quitting smoking could mean that you do not get the nicotine fix you desire from vaping and for a lot of people that leads them straight back to tobacco. If you find yourself still craving cigarettes or vaping obsessively for long periods of time it could be that you are not getting the nicotine that you are accustomed to and should consider stepping up your nicotine a bit.

The reverse may be true if you find that vaping leaves you light headed or nauseous. Although the brain is pretty good at self regulating and you'll normally not have the desire to pick up your vape if you've already had too much nicotine, sometimes people continue to vape regardless and nausea could be a sign that you are vaping with too much nicotine and should drop down a level.

Your end goal with vaping is entirely up to you. Some people use vaping as a temporary measure to cease smoking tobacco and gradually wind down their dependence on nicotine to zero until they don't even need to vape anymore. Others step down their nicotine level to a comfortable zone and continue vaping permanently.

Another factor you must consider when choosing the nicotine strength of your e-liquid is the device that you are using and how you vape. If you enjoy direct-to-lung style vaping using a sub-ohm setup, you will be vaporizing and consuming considerably more e-liquid than someone vaping mouth-to-lung on a higher resistance, lower power device and therefore you should use a much lower concentration of nicotine to maintain the same intake levels.

Tanks

When you start moving up from basic all-in-one devices to the more advanced mods you need to decide on which tank to use.

Some mods are sold as a standalone units whereas others are sold as part of a kit and include a tank. Almost all mods, including those sold as a kit, are capable of supporting a wide variety of different tanks.

A tank is a cylindrical device that that generally consists of a glass casing to house the e-liquid and an atomizer. At the base of the tank you will find a standard connector known as a 510 connector for attaching the tank onto a mod. Nearly all tanks and mods on the market use the standard 510 connector, meaning you are free to mix and match using a variety of different brands. At the top of the tank is a mouthpiece that is used to inhale the vapor from the tank.

There are a great deal of different types of tanks on the market, each with very differing features and uses and there are numerous things to take into account when considering what type of tank is suitable for you.

Airflow

One of the most important design considerations for a tank is the airflow. How air is drawn into the device, passes over your heated coils and eventually gets sucked upwards into your mouth can have a tremendous impact on the overall vaping experience. Even small adjustments to the amount or direction of airflow can completely change the density of vapor and the intensity of flavor that you can get from your tank

The main factor to consider relating to airflow is the quantity of air that can pass through the tank and this is largely influenced by your vaping style. We've already discussed different vaping styles that suit different people, from mouth-to-lung to direct-lung vaping. Vapers who prefer a mouth-to-lung experience will need to choose a tank that offers a more restrictive airflow, that is to say, that less airflow passes through the tank and there is a notable resistance when you pull on the device. This is much the same as pulling on a regular tobacco cigarette.

Those who opt to vape direct-to-lung however have the opposite requirement and usually need a tank that has large air inlets in order to be able to breath in larger amounts of air when they vape.

Most modern tanks offer an adjustable airflow option to open or close the air inlets incrementally, however different tanks will have different airflow capacity when the inlets are opened up all the way and for some this might be too restrictive for direct-lung vaping. When reading or watching reviews of tanks on the marketplace you will often see that they have been engineered to cater for one specific style.

The placement of air inlets also has a huge impact on the resulting vaping experience. Many tanks have air inlets at the base of the unit that allows air to be drawn in very close to the coils, while others have top airflow systems where air is drawn from the top, down to the base of the coil and then up again through the center shaft of the tank to your mouth. All of the varying airflow options that we find with modern day tanks have pros and cons, and you may have to try and few different varieties before deciding on what kind of airflow suits your personal vaping preference.

Mouthpiece

A crucial but often overlooked part of a tank is the mouthpiece that fits onto the top. Mouthpieces, or drip tips as they are sometimes known, come in a huge variety of shapes and sizes and can be made out of several different materials.

The majority of higher end, advanced tanks on the marketplace come with a mouthpiece included or already installed onto the tank however they are replaceable and can easily be removed and substituted for a different type of mouthpiece.

Generally speaking, mouthpieces are either 510 or 810, this denotes the diameter of the base of the drip tip that you insert into the top of your tank. 510 mouthpieces have a slightly narrower opening than most 810 types.

Manufacturers of tanks are acutely aware of the varying preferences of their users so a lot of modern tanks from good brands will contain an adapter inside the box to enable you to use either a 510 or an 810 sized mouthpiece.

The size and shape of the mouthpiece not only defines how comfortable it is to use, but also the airflow that passes from the tank into your mouth. As we've already discussed, airflow is a key consideration when vaping. A lot of mouth-to-lung style vapers will opt for a mouthpiece that is thin at the tip, allowing for a restricted pull with plenty of air resistance. Other mouthpieces cater more for direct-lung vapers with large open tips capable of passing lots of air for hard, unrestricted pulls.

Mouthpieces are also made out of a variety of different materials from resins, plastic, metal and even glass. Different materials provide a different sensation on your lips and mouth when using them and it's entirely down to a vapers preference which type they prefer. Different materials also conduct heat very differently and some mouthpieces are made of resins which are more suitable to be used on tanks that are designed at very high wattage to stop the heat from the tank traveling up to your lips.

Refilling and Capacity

Tanks offer a variety of different ways to be able to top up your e-liquid. In the case of most modern tanks you need to unscrew part of the tank to reveal the reservoir inlet in order to add more liquid. The majority of tanks today are top-fill tanks, meaning that you unscrew or flip open the top section along with the mouthpiece in order to add liquid. There are some models however known as bottom-fill tanks that you must unscrew the base of the tank, keeping the tank upside down, to access the inlet. My preference is always for top-fill tanks, as they can be opened without having to unscrew and disconnect the tank from the mod making topping up your e-liquid much easier.

There is a small argument to be made for bottom fill tanks. Tanks control the rate in which liquid can be passed through to the wick and coil by nature of a vacuum within the liquid reservoir. When you open a top-fill tank, any liquid left in the reservoir will be able to flow quicker into the coil because whilst the lid is open there is no vacuum holding the liquid back. In reality however I find that so long as I top up reasonably quickly and don't leave the top open for extended periods of time this is rarely a problem and still better than the inconvenience of using a bottom-fill tank.

The last characteristic of a tank worth mentioning capacity – tanks can hold anywhere from one or two milliliters of liquid, up to seven or eight for larger units. Recent legislation in Europe requires all tanks to hold a maximum of two millimeters of liquid, although larger tanks are still very commonplace in other countries in the world.

If you are vaping at higher wattages direct to lung you are likely to consume considerable amounts of e-liquid, so a tank with a limited capacity will mean constant refilling, so this is a notable consideration.

So as you can see, although many tanks may look the same at first glance, there are many subtle factors that can change the overall vaping experience and understanding what to look for in a new tank will hopefully guide you into finding a tank that fits your vaping preference perfectly.

Rebuildable Atomizers

Vaping can start out as a simple new activity that replaces smoking of tobacco, and for some people over time it can start developing into a hobby. As my interest in vaping grew, I started viewing videos online of the latest tanks and mods and soon started to grow a collection of different vaping paraphernalia and e-liquids. It was however with one discovery that my interest crossed the line into a full blown hobby, and that discovery was for me, rebuildable atomizers.

With a traditional tank system, you place a factory made atomizer containing a coil inside the tank. These types of atomizers are very easy to work with, when your coil is at the end of its natural life or burns out, you simply open your tank, unscrew the small self-contained atomizer unit and replace it with a new one. This type of atomizer is known as a *drop in* coil. With a rebuildable system however there are no factory made atomizers, you manually install the coil wire and wicking cotton yourself.

The world of rebuildable systems is for more advanced vapers, although it's relatively easy to get into when you've been vaping for a while and you are familiar with how electronic cigarettes work.

The most common type of rebuildable is a rebuildable tank atomizer, often referred to as an RTA. An RTA looks very similar to a regular tank, it has the same cylindrical shape, and the same 510 connector pin found on any other tank. The difference can be seen when you dis-assemble it. Most RTAs allow you to unscrew the main section of the tank from the base. When the base is exposed you'll find a platform containing a system of small holes and screws and often has channels that lead down into a well or chamber where a small amount of e-liquid can sit. This platform is called the *build deck*. The build deck provides connection points between the positive and negative terminals of the circuit within the device.

In order to use an RTA you need to install a wrapped piece of wire, the coil, between these positive and negative points that will complete the circuit when you fire your device. A lot of RTAs support more than one coil placement, dual coil RTAs are commonplace. The process of installing the coils is what is referred to in the rebuildable world as *building.*

Once a coil has been successfully installed on the build deck, the second step is to add a cotton based wicking material to soak up the e-liquid that you'll eventually add into the tank. This second stage to preparing a rebuildable atomizer is what we call *wicking.*

Constructing a rebuildable atomizer is an advanced form of vaping. You are responsible for connecting the positive and negative ends of a circuit that will pull current from your battery. If you do not have a solid understanding of battery safety, ohms and amperage it is not recommended. Regulated mods have circuitry between your battery and your coil that provides many levels of protection, including short circuit protection that make building and using rebuildable atomizers safer in the event that you mistakenly introduce a bad build. Mechanical mods however do not offer any safety features, if you install a coil that places too much stress on the battery or it connects with another part of the build deck and creates a short circuit, you could destroy your device and risk serious personal injury. **Inexperienced vapers should not attempt to construct a rebuildable atomizer for use on a mechanical mod.** We will discuss battery safety later in this book, but this is a point that needs to be highlighted.

Building

Building is much more than just placing a wire into two screw holes. Building starts with selecting the type of coil that you want to run. Coils can be bought pre-wrapped to a specific size and length and can be made out of a variety of different metals, all of which have different qualities depending on how you like to vape and the characteristics of your RTA.

As well as pre-wrapped coils, you can also buy spools of wire in the material and gauge that you need and wrap them into coils yourself.

Wrapping your own coils may seem overly complicated but with a few basic tools and after a couple of attempts following one of the many guides available online, you'll soon find that it's pretty simple, and gives you the ultimate level of finite control over how to fine tune your coils to your preference.

You can build your own coil by using a regular screwdriver of approximately 2.5mm in diameter. Simply place the coil wire against the screw driver and wrap the wire around several times until you have a wrapped coil resembling a closed spring. Coil legs, the straight wire on both ends of the wrapped coil can then be cut to the desired size using wire cutters.

Although a regular screwdriver can do the trick, many prefer to use a tool called a *coil jig*. With a coil jig you select your desired diameter of your final coil, place one end of the wire into a small hole and hold it in place. The coil can be wrapped much more easily with a cap that you rotate. It's considerably easier than trying to wrap a coil by pulling it around a screwdriver with your fingers.

When building your own coils there are several things to consider, beginning with the type of wire to use.

Coil wire can be made out of several types of metal. One of the more common materials used for wire construction is Kanthal. This type of wire makes coils that are perfect for people getting into rebuildable atomizers and vape in standard wattage mode.

For the more adventurous vaper there are other coil wires such as stainless steel or nichrome that can be used with more advanced forms of vaping such as temperature controlled mode. Other more exotic coil wires can be found that combine two or more different wires together, such as the well known Clapton coils that are made of a base wire wrapped with a much thinner wire tightly wrapped around it.

The gauge of the wire is basically a unit of measuring the diameter of the wire. Lower gauge wires result in lower resistance in your final build as they are thicker than higher gauge wires. A 23 gauge wire will result in a much lower resistance than a thinner 30 gauge wire.

The gauge and material of your coil wire help determine what the resistance your coil will reach. There are two remaining controllable factors that will also affect this. The diameter of the coil itself when wrapped and the number of wraps that make up the coil.

When building a coil you should be aiming for a target resistance that you wish to end up with. Bear in mind that when dealing with more than one coil the resistance is shared. When building with identical coils, you need to divide the target resistance of each coil by the number of coils to get an accurate idea of what resistance your final build will be. That means, if you are building for a dual coil RTA and each of your coils has a resistance of 0.4Ω, because you have two coils your final resistance on your device will be around 0.2Ω.

With so many factors affecting the final resistance of a coil it may seem like a science to determine an accurate outcome, and it is. Fortunately there are tools which vapers rely on to take away some of the complicated mathematics out of it. The most popular tool for building coils is the calculator available on *steamengine.org*. Simply enter in that parameters of your build, the wire type and gauge, the diameter of the coil that you wish to build, and the desired resistance that you are aiming for and the calculator will do the maths and tell you how many wraps you need to achieve it.

Once you have built and installed your coils it's necessary to make sure they heat up properly. This can be done by dry firing the device at a medium power setting and watching how the coils glow as they get hot.

A new coil will often not glow evenly and contain visible hot spots that need to be eliminated. A gentle strumming with a pair of tweezers will help to remove hot spots in your coils. Unless you have ceramic tweezers you should never strum the coils whilst firing them as you could create a short circuit through the metallic ends.

After strumming and dry firing your coils they should glow evenly from the middle of the coil spreading outwards, and if you are installing two coils they should glow evenly between them.

Wicking

After building and installing your coil into your RTA you need to add a wicking material, usually cotton, through your coil and into the wells that will draw in the e-liquid to your coil.

Every RTA is wicked slightly differently to achieve optimum performance, but the basics involve taking a strip of cotton ensuring that it is of the correct density, compressing it slightly so it passes through the center of your coil. Determining the correct amount of cotton to thread through your coil can be a bit of a fine art and can only really be learned through trial and error. You should aim for the cotton to pass through the coil with a little resistance, but not so much that your coils move or you damage the cotton trying to drag it through. Similarly, you don't want it too loose either, if you can pull the cotton through with no resistance at all and it simply slides through with no effort, then you probably don't have enough cotton. Cotton packed too tightly will mean that the liquid cannot soak into the center of the coil effectively enough and you risk burnt and dry hits as the cotton will be too dry. If the cotton is too lose it will not bind with the coils properly and you'll likely have a rather disappointing result.

Getting the right balance takes a little time. I have a lot of experience with rebuildable atomizers and even I misjudge my cotton sometimes and have to pull it all out and start again, it happens to us all.

Finally, once your cotton is securely in place threaded through your coil you'll need to trim either end of the wick before placing each end inside the well where it will come into contact with the e-liquid and draw it inwards.   The amount of cotton to trim is entirely dependent on the design of the RTA. Some devices have large deep wells that require long cotton tails, others are shallow with small wicking channels that need a minimum amount of cotton.

Once the wick is in place it is vitally important to prime the cotton with your e-juice and ensure it is well soaked with no dry parts touching the coils before firing the coil. Once you've primed the wick by dripping small amounts of liquid on all parts of the cotton, the tank can be fully assembled and e-liquid added to the reservoir. The RTA is now ready to vape.

There are a multitude of tutorial videos on the Internet showing how to wick nearly any type of RTA on the market. It only takes a little experimentation to find the right wicking method for your RTA.

Dripping with an RDA

Dripping is described by some to be the ultimate vaping experience. It's rare that someone starts dripping from day one of being a vaper, it's often a practice that is arrived at after considerable time getting familiar with the various concepts of vaping.

Dripping is basically using a device similar to a tank, but instead of topping up a reservoir containing several millimeters of liquid to be slowly absorbed into the coil over time, you simply drip your liquid directly onto the wicking materials or coil, and vape.

Dripping is normally done using a rebuildable dripping atomizer, or RDA. Although similar to an RTA, an RDA is often distinguishable by being slightly shorter and doesn't have a glass outer casing since there is no reservoir to store e-liquid. An RDA has at its base a build deck very similar to one that you'll find on an RTA. On top of the build deck normally sits a removable middle section, a cylindrical tube with air inlets cut into it. Finally there is a top cap that sits on top of the middle section where the mouthpiece is attached.

RDAs are normally dis-assembled simply by pulling off the top cap and middle section, there is rarely much to unscrew. You can add more e-liquid to an RDA by pulling off the top cap and dripping liquid down directly onto the wicks. Some RDAs are designed to easily drip through the mouthpiece without removing the top cap at all.

Once the cotton is soaked, you can vape. However, because there isn't a reservoir of liquid to provide more liquid to the wicking process over time, you will not be able to vape for as long as you can with an RTA before having to refill it again. Most RDAs will offer about six or seven good pulls before you notice the flavor and cloud density dulling and at that point you should drip some more liquid into your device to avoid the cotton drying out completely and burning.

Whilst dripping requires more constant effort, regularly adding more liquid every few pulls, most people who drip claim that the flavor quality and density of the vapor produced is far superior to any other form of vaping.

Of course, dripping is not suitable for all scenarios. If you vape while driving for example it would not be feasible to have to pull over to the side of the road every six puffs in order to drip more liquid into your device, so regular tanks or RTAs still have a place in a vapers arsenal as they can be more convenient.

Although dripping is considered one of the more advanced forms of vaping, once you are familiar with working with an RTA, making the transition to a dripping atomizer is relatively easy. The build deck on an RDA is very similar. Building coils for an RDA is almost an identical process to an RTA. Wicking an RDA involves a little understanding of the differences. With an RTA you normally trim your cotton to place it into wicking channels to make contact with the reservoir of liquid that will feed into it, with an RDA there is normally a small well either side of your coil that you simply stuff your cotton into.

Most people find dripping atomizers considerably easier to wick as they don't require so much finessing to ensure the optimal wicking process from a tank.

Squonking

As vaping methods get more bizarre and interesting, so do the names that get given to them. Squonking certainly fits that description.

Squonking is a relatively new arrival in mainstream vaping, but has proven popular with a lot of people. Whilst RDAs are considered the best form of vaping, they come at the expense of convenience as you have to constantly refill your device. Squonk systems aim to solve this by making it easier to keep your wicks primed with liquid by simply pressing a button rather than manually dripping liquid from a bottle.

A squonk mod, like a regular mod contains a battery for powering the device but also houses a bottle of e-liquid inside the device itself. When activated, liquid can be pushed up through the pin that connects the mod to the RDA that sits on top of it, soaking the wicks to enable you to continue vaping.

In order to use a squonk mod you need an RDA that is compatible. The liquid is passed from the mod to the RDA via a small hole in the 510 connector pin that is also used to feed power to the coil. A lot of newer RDAs now come with a removable 510 connector pin and a replacement one that has a hole suitable for use with a squonk mod.

Becoming a Hobby

As you can see, there is a lot to learn, and do, when you start down the road of rebuildable atomizers whether they be drippers or tanks. It's not for everyone, if you are simply looking for a smoking alternative with the minimal of effort and maintenance then you should stick with pre-made drop in coils in a a medium range setup, there's nothing wrong with that.

But if you do decide to embark on rebuildable devices, it can eventually turn into quite a rewarding hobby. Experimenting with different build types, different wires, different wicking materials can open up your vaping experience to many new levels.

Maybe not everyone will understand your new hobby, but, if like me, when you spend your Sunday mornings sipping coffee on your patio and rebuilding your RDAs for pleasure, your spouse looks at you like you're mad, just remember, you're not smoking, so who cares?

Batteries and Safety

If you talk to enough people about vaping eventually the subject will come up of exploding electronic cigarettes and how dangerous vaping is. We've all seen the news articles recounting how some unfortunate people have received quite horrific injuries attributed to using electronic cigarettes and in one recent case in the United States there was a tragic fatality.

A lot of media outlets seize upon the opportunity to write sensationalist articles reporting about exploding e-cigarettes, not many take the time to fully research and report the facts. This leaves a lot of people with the belief that if they start vaping they risk blowing their teeth out with every puff they take. This misplaced fear often means they'll continue smoking, an activity very likely to shorten their life. There lies the irony.

As a community, vapers are very concerned with keeping people safe, and we are always deeply troubled to hear a case of someone who has been injured or even killed in an activity related to vaping. We also consider it hugely important to educate people about the facts of vaping safety, not only to protect the integrity of vaping from misinformation so people who smoke tobacco are not discouraged from taking up vaping instead, but also to ensure that others don't have the same experience.

The only component of an electronic cigarette capable of failure in a remotely catastrophic way is the battery used to power the device. Electronic cigarettes use high drain lithium-ion batteries to provide the power needed to heat your coils.

Whilst a lot of entry level devices have internally hosted non-removable batteries, most of the more advanced mods use external batteries. The vast majority of external battery power mods use a standard of battery known as *18650*.

The numbers given to a battery normally refer to its size and shape – in the case of 18650 it denotes that the cell is 18 millimeters wide and 65 millimeters tall.

Whilst other less common battery sizes are used in some vaping mods, such as 26650 cells, the chemistry used internally inside the battery and the steps you need to ensure that you use and care for your battery safely remain the same.

Batteries used in vaping are typically made for electronics manufacturers and are intended for use inside devices such as laptops or grouped together to form battery packs to provide power for high demand products such as electric bikes. Vaping is not the only popular personal use for these types of batteries, they have been used for years by flashlight enthusiast.

Battery Voltage

Batteries are made with what is called a nominal voltage. In the case of most batteries that we use for vaping, the nominal voltage is 3.6-3.7V.

The voltage of a battery is not a constant however, a fully charged battery starts at a voltage much higher than the nominal voltage and decreases over time as you draw power from it.

The specifications of a particular type of battery include a fully charged voltage limit, usually 4.2V for the standard 18650 cells that are commonplace in vaping. It is very important that you never charge a battery beyond the recommended fully charged voltage or you could risk serious damage to the battery resulting in fire or personal injury. A good charging device for your batteries should automatically cut off charging at or slightly below this limit, but they should still be monitored and not left unattended.

As you continue to use a battery, the voltage will slowly decrease. The speed in which batteries experience this voltage drop off varies, and time and much use you may notice that batteries lose voltage at a much quicker rate than they used to. This is normally a sign that the battery is coming to the end of its useful life and you should safely dispose of the battery. Most good quality batteries will run for a year or two of every day vaping before an increase in voltage drop off time is notable.

Just as it is important that you do not overcharge your batteries, it is also very important that the voltage does not fall too low. Letting the voltage of a battery fall to 3.0V might shorten the batteries useful life, and you should never let a battery fall anywhere near 2.5V or below or you could irreparably damage the battery.

As we will discuss more later, regulated mods have a cut off point where they will refuse to fire if the battery voltage drops to a certain point, normally 3.2V. The battery level indicator that many mods have will usually give you the percentage of available power before cut off, rather than the entire capacity of the battery, zero percent being 3.2V.

Users of regulated mods therefore do not need to worry too much about ensuring batteries are not depleted too low, however for those with mechanical mods, there is no protection against draining a battery to critical levels, and as we will see later on in this chapter, doing so could risk serious damage.

Understanding mAhs and Amps

There are two important characteristics of a battery. The capacity of the battery measured in milliamp hours and represented as a number followed by *mAh*. This number determines how much charge the battery can hold, determining how long it will last before needing to be recharged. Typical high end batteries used in vaping will be in the region of 2000-3000mAh.

It's impossible to say purely based on the batteries capacity how long it will last when using it to vape, as this will vary wildly depending on the amps drawn from the battery when you fire your mod.

Using your device at higher wattages will result in more power being drained from the battery. This drain is measured in amps, represented by the letter *A* and is referred to as a *CDR*, or, *continuous discharge rate.*

It is very important that you know the continuous discharge rating of the battery that you are using and understand how to avoid drawing more amps from the battery than it is rated for. Pushing a battery beyond its continuous discharge rating could cause the battery to fail resulting in it venting hot gases and possibly catching fire.

Calculating amperage

With mechanical mod where there is no electronic circuitry to control the power levels, the amount of power drawn from the battery is dependent on the resistance of the coil installed in the atomizer. The lower the resistance, the higher the power drain on the battery will be. When using mechanical mods therefore it's vital to understand the principles of *Ohms Law.*

Ohms law is a small set of calculations to determine what the battery drain will be based on the voltage of the battery and the resistance of the coil.

Regulated mods however are very different, since there is a circuit board in between the battery and the coil that controls the amount of power flowing through the circuit that determines the draw on the battery.

To calculate the amperage drawn from a battery when using a regulated mod you simply take the wattage level that your device is set to and divide by the voltage of the battery.

Since most vaping batteries have a fully charged voltage of 4.2V that slowly drops over time as you use your device, the amperage drawn from the battery will start off lower and slowly rise. When calculating safe vaping limits you should work out your amperage based on the lowest voltage level of your battery. Most modern regulated mods have an automatic cut off point and will not allow you to completely deplete the battery, the battery indicator on a regulated mod normally represents the amount of power left within the cut off range, not the amount of battery charge in total. For most regulated single battery mods this cut off point is

3.2V. So in order to determine the amount of amps draining from your battery you should divide the number of watts by 3.2, it is also advisable to add a ten percent buffer zone to account for small inaccuracies with the exact wattage your device uses.

$$amps = (\,watts\,/\,3.2\,)\,/\,0.9$$

So if you are vaping with your mod set to 35W, you divide this by 3.2 and further divide the result by 0.9 to account for the ten percent head room and you can determine that you are draining your battery at 12A when the battery is close to its cut off point, which will be the maximum draw. Therefore you should ensure that your batteries have a CDR rating of 12A or above in order to ensure that you are vaping safely.

When using a regulated device that runs on more than one battery it's important to note that the load on the batteries will be shared. When performing the above calculations you should factor in 3.2V for each battery that your device contains. For example, a dual battery regulated mod vaping at 35W would be just over 6A on each battery, roughly half of the total drain on a single battery mod. This is because we now have 6.4V of current as opposed to 3.2V. The calculations used to determine the amps per battery are the same;

$$(35w / \mathbf{6.4v}) / 0.9 = 6.07A$$

Ohm's Law

Ohm's Law is a series of calculations that use three underpinning factors of current (amps), voltage and resistance. Normally using two of these to determine the third.

When spending any amount of time on vaping forums you will come across advice stating the importance of understanding Ohm's Law. In vaping, we use Ohm's Law determine the amperage drawn from the battery based on the voltage and resistance of the coil. What is poorly understood however is that for users of regulated devices Ohm's Law has no real significance whatsoever, because we are using electronic circuit boards with chips to regulate the amount of power that the coils are fired at by specifying the wattage level, the amp drain on the battery is a controllable factor and can be worked out with the simple calculations above.

When using a regulated mod, the resistance of the coil is largely unimportant from a battery safety point of view.

The only consideration you must take into account is that for very low resistance builds you are likely going to need to fire your device at a higher power setting in order to be able to heat the coils efficiently enough to provide a satisfying vape and you should make sure that the power level you vape at will result in a battery load thats within the continuous discharge rate limit of your battery.

For users of mechanical mods however, Ohm's Law is of critical importance.

With a mechanical mod, the resistance of the coil is the only thing that controls the power that is pulled from the battery. Using a coil with a very low resistance in a mech mod could result in pulling more amperage than your battery is rated for and this could potentially stress the battery beyond its limits.

Testing and verifying the resistance of a coil is very important when using a mechanical mod as we use the resistance to determine the drain from the battery.

When vaping with a mechanical mod you can work out the amp drain on the battery by using the two known factors of voltage and resistance to work out the amps that will be drawn from the battery. We do this by simply taking the voltage and dividing it by the resistance of the coil. So if we have a fully charged battery at 4.2V and a single coil reading 0.4Ω we can use these two measurements to determine the amps that will be drawn from the battery

$$4.2V / 0.4Ω = 10.5A$$

As you continue vaping however the voltage of your battery will slowly decrease meaning the amp draw will also fall, if we replace 4.2V with 3.7V, the nominal voltage of an 18650 battery, we see that the draw on the battery falls to 9.2A.

As you can see, the calculations we use on a mechanical mod are very different to those relevant for a regulated device.

Since mechanical mods have no circuitry or chips, that means they are also incapable of monitoring battery capacity, there is no automatic cut off with a mechanical mod and it's entirely up to the user to stop using a battery before it discharges to an unrecommended level that could seriously affect the performance of the battery.

Battery re-wraps

There are very few companies that can successfully manufacture high drain lithium-ion batteries that offer a sizable capacity with a high enough CDR rating for modern vaping. The science and logistics behind making these batteries is extensive, and expensive. A select few electronics companies including Sony, LG and Samsung have been dominating this space for many years now. The only real newcomer to this scene in recent times has come in the form of Elon Musk investing substantial amounts of money to develop the *"Gigafactories"* that produce lithium-ion based batteries that power, among other things, Tesla electric vehicles.

With the barrier to entry set so high, you may wonder why you regularly see lithium-ion batteries being branded and sold by little known vaping companies.

The reality is that a lot of smaller companies offering their own brand batteries are simply buying batches of batteries from the main manufacturers and replacing the wrapping for one that has their own branding and re-selling them.

Most of the key manufacturers will produce large batches of batteries, and similarly to fine wine producers, they will often separate the final products into bins, depending on the quality of the final battery. The bins of the highest quality will normally be sold to major electronics manufacturers and used in consumer products such as laptops and tablets. The lesser quality bins are often sold on to companies who re-wrap and resell them.

The real issue arises when the companies that buy, re-wrap and resell the battery inflate the continuous discharge rating of the battery. As vaping has become big business and many vapers are always looking to get more power out of their batteries to fire sub-ohm coils, battery re-sellers see rating batteries with very high amp limits as a way to increase sales.

Not all 18650 batteries are suitable for modern vaping, some offer as little as 5A continuous discharge rating but can be sold in the marketplace by unscrupulous re-wrap vendors claiming a discharge limit of 20A or more. Placing a 20A load on a battery only rated to 5A is potentially very dangerous.

Not all re-wrapped battery distributors partake in this practice, but if you are unsure it is always wise to buy top brand batteries from a supplier that you trust.

Battery Mooch

The world of vaping batteries can be confusing, with numerous models claiming different capacities and continuous discharge ratings with varying degrees of truthfulness it can be difficult to know if you are vaping safely within the limits of your batteries or not. Thankfully, the vaping community has *Battery Mooch*. Mooch is the online moniker of a man that has dedicated considerable amounts of time testing and rating nearly every common vaping battery on the market with measured capacity and continuous discharge ratings that he regularly publishes online and his research and efforts are well trusted, and appreciated by the vaping community. Mooch has a blog hosted on the ECF forum, you can find the website address at the end of this book.

Battery Safety Tips

We've looked at how to ensure that the battery that you use is appropriate for the type and power of your device to ensure that batteries are not placed under undue stress, which can lead to issues that result in injury. Many reported cases of accidents related to vaping however result from carelessness in the storage or charging of batteries.

It's important to understand that the batteries that we use for vaping are high powered cells, and furthermore most do not contain any kind of protection circuitry to prevent a hard short.

A battery hard short occurs when the positive and negative ends of the battery come into contact with each other via a conductive material, that contact can quickly lead to the battery heating up at an exponential rate and entering a state known as *thermal runaway* where the heat and pressure builds up too quickly and the battery splits open and furiously vents hot gas.

In some devices, particularly cylindrical mechanical mods with inadequate ventilation this can lead to the creation of so much pressure that the device itself explodes, much like how a pipe bomb operates.

It's these highly unfortunate, and very rare accidents that often make headline news and focus peoples attention away from the huge health benefits of vaping as an alternative to tobacco, and fill potential new vapers with fear of exploding vape pens.

The reality is that there are simple steps you can take to ensure that your vaping experience is as safe as making a call on your smart phone.

Battery Storage

As we've already discussed, when the positive and negative ends of a battery connect via a conductive material, we can create a hard short resulting in catastrophic battery failure.

Many reported cases of injury are not the result of using an electronic cigarette, but of batteries going into thermal runaway after a short created by keys or other metallic objects inside a pocket or bag.

You should **never** store or carry loose batteries. Plastic battery cases made especially for 18650 and other sized vaping batteries are available online and in most good vaping shops and rarely cost more then $1-$2, a very small investment to ensure your personal safety.

When a battery is not installed inside your mod, or in your charger, it should always be in a closed plastic case.

Charging

If you have replaceable batteries for your mod you should invest in an external charger from a recommended and well trusted brand. Many mods have a USB connection that enables you to charge the batteries whilst the batteries are in the device.

Overcharging a battery is a well known cause of battery failures resulting in fire and explosion, top brand external battery chargers usually have considerably more failsafe and monitoring features to ensure safe battery charging.

Never leave batteries charging unattended or for extended periods of time.

The 18650 batteries that we use for vaping should never be charged beyond their recommended limit, which is normally 4.2V and most external battery chargers will automatically cut off charging slightly below this point. As a further precautionary measure you could use a multimeter to ensure that your charger is performing correctly and safely by measuring the battery voltage when removed from the charger.

Damaged Batteries

Another common reason for battery failure is physical damage to the battery. Batteries should be retired and disposed of if they show any sign of physical damage such as dents.

It's also very important to check the plastic wrapping of your batteries to make sure they are in tact and have no nicks or tears.   We have already discussed the importance of not allowing any conductive object to create a connection between the positive and negative parts of a battery.   It is not just the two ends of the battery that you should be concerned about.   The positive area of a battery is the small disc located in the center of the top end of the cell, everything else on the battery including the outer part of the top section and the entire body of the battery is the negative terminal. All but the bottom exposed part of the battery should be covered in a non-conductive plastic wrap. If this wrap is even slightly torn you may expose part of the metal that makes up the negative part of the battery and risk accidentally short circuiting your battery if it comes into contact with other conductive objects.

This is especially true if the battery wrap is torn towards the top of the battery, you could easily expose negative parts of the battery that are normally covered by a small plastic ring and are mere millimeters away from the positive terminal.   This could very easily lead to a creating a hard short inside your device or when inserting or removing it from your charger. You should always briefly inspect your batteries and their wrappers every time you use them.

If a battery wrap is in any way damaged it can easily be re-wrapped. Battery wraps can be purchased from most good vaping stores and can be applied to a stripped battery using just a hair dryer. Some vaping stores will also perform this service for you if you are unsure of how to do it safely.

Disposal of Batteries

Eventually, batteries do reach the end of their useful life and need to be disposed of. Remember that just because a battery is no longer suitable for vaping, it's still highly likely that the battery contains enough voltage to hard short if it comes into contact with other conductive objects. Furthermore, all batteries contain chemistry that is highly toxic to the environment if discarded in a way whereby they can contaminate ground soil or water.

Never dispose of batteries in your regular household refuse. Battery recycling facilities are available in a variety of places, and many vape shops also offer this service free of charge.

For safety reasons, I recommend that you always completely cover both the positive and negative ends of the battery with non-conductive electrical tape and then further wrapping them in a freezer bag to prevent other items from easily nicking the wrapping. This ensures that your batteries can be transported safely from the collection point to the plant.

Conclusion

When you pull the curtain back and look behind the headlines and news articles on exploding vaping devices, we see that the vast majority of these unfortunate incidents are down to user error in one way or another. Most accidents that result in injury can be attributed to users of mechanical mods who have insufficient understanding of how to operate them safely and batteries stored in pockets or bags in an unsafe way. The third most common reported cause of battery failure is overcharging.

No battery, especially lithium-ion based batteries, are one hundred percent safe. But with some basic knowledge and common sense there is no reason why you should be any more concerned about safety when vaping as you would be using your mobile phone or laptop.

Final Thoughts

A Call to Action

Vaping has given me a great deal. It has been, and continues to be a fun and interesting pastime that eventually lead me to write a book about it. But above all, for me and for so many people like me, it has allowed me to defeat a demon that beforehand seemed impossible, to stand up to, and stub out my smoking habit once and for all and in doing so, provided me with the opportunity to make sure my little boy has his daddy for as many years as possible.

The huge surge in popularity over recent years now has sparked debate among lawmakers over how and if to regulate the industry.

While scientific bodies are now weighing in, mostly with positive evidence suggesting that vaping is considerably less harmful than smoking, the fact that vaping is a mere decade old and some of the more recent types of devices have only been around for two or three years, means that progress is slow. Some government bodies have been quick to jump the gun and impose overly restrictive laws around vaping concerning themselves with the perceived risk rather than acknowledging that the vaping revolution is saving potentially millions of lives.

Some countries such as Argentina and Thailand have placed an outright ban on all forms of vaping, whilst others have proceeded more cautiously aligning vaping with existing tobacco smoking laws governing where they can be used.

In the US the Federal Drugs Administration (FDA) have recently introduced a range of far sweeping proposals that many consider heavy handed and unnecessary, including stringent requirements on manufacturers making it prohibitively expensive for smaller vaping companies to compete and a complete ban on all flavored liquids.

The FDA seems to be basing many of its decisions on a presumption that vaping is a gateway to tobacco smoking for children and teenagers, a viewpoint that more recent studies in the UK refute. The rise in use of the JUUL vaping pod in schools and colleges is seen as the catalyst for the action with several anti smoking groups queuing up to support tough legislation.

In Europe, we've seen the harshest blow yet to vaping in the form of the Tobacco Products Directive (TPD) which alongside tobacco products also introduces a wide range of restrictions around vaping.

The TPD legislation makes it illegal to sell any liquid containing nicotine in quantities greater than 10ml. It also places a cap of 20mg/ml of nicotine for any liquid, meaning some ex-smokers who rely on high strength nicotine of 24mg/ml or above to keep them from smoking are now struggling under the new laws.

TPD also places a range of restrictions on vaping hardware manufacturers, most notably that tanks must hold a maximum of 2ml of liquid.

Both the FDA proposals in the US and the TPD which is now law in Europe have drawn heavy criticism from the vaping community and from some scientific and medical bodies.

As government departments continue to consider regulations there is rife speculation that lobbying organizations supporting global tobacco companies are unduly influencing legislation and that tax collected from tobacco products is considered under threat as more people switch to vaping.

Cigarette smoking is by far the leading cause of preventable death. Millions of ex-smokers would still be smoking today if they hadn't made the switch to vaping, which is widely believed to be up to ninety-five percent safer than the tobacco alternative. It's hard to see how regulating vaping to the point that in some places it's easier and cheaper to buy tobacco cigarettes than it is to vape is in any way in the interests of public health.

If this matters to you, there are numerous ways to make your voice heard. One of the best known vaping advocacy groups is the Consumer Advocates for Smoke Free Alternatives Association (CASAA). They do lots of work on behalf of the vaping community trying to positively influence and educate people to ensure the future of vaping. You can get involved at their website, *casaa.org*.

ECF Forum

There are many forums and groups online to find out more about vaping and ask questions. One of the largest is the E-Cigarette Forum (ECF) at _www.e-cigarette-forum.com_.

The ECF forum is well run and have discussion groups from absolute beginners to the more advanced forms of vaping. The community that has built around the forum is welcoming and friendly and always keen to help people with their vaping questions, or simply congratulate you on your path to a smoke free life.

ECF is also the home of the battery blog written by Mooch, where detailed and reliable test results for vaping batteries are published.

I would like to extend special acknowledgment and thanks to ECF who not only have provided me with many answers to my questions as I embarked on my own vaping journey but were also a source of inspiration for writing this book

Happy Vaping

I hope you found the contents of this book interesting and helpful, if you have suggestions or corrections please let me know by contacting me. The vaping world changes so rapidly, I will try and update this book with the latest future developments so please keep checking in.

Follow me on Twitter at @crayfishx

Get news and updates on this book at *vapingbook.info*

www.ingramcontent.com/pod-product-compliance
Lightning Source LLC
Chambersburg PA
CBHW031413250726
48656CB00002B/657